AF075827

How to feel fabulous the alkaline way

EMMA LEHANE

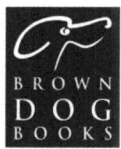

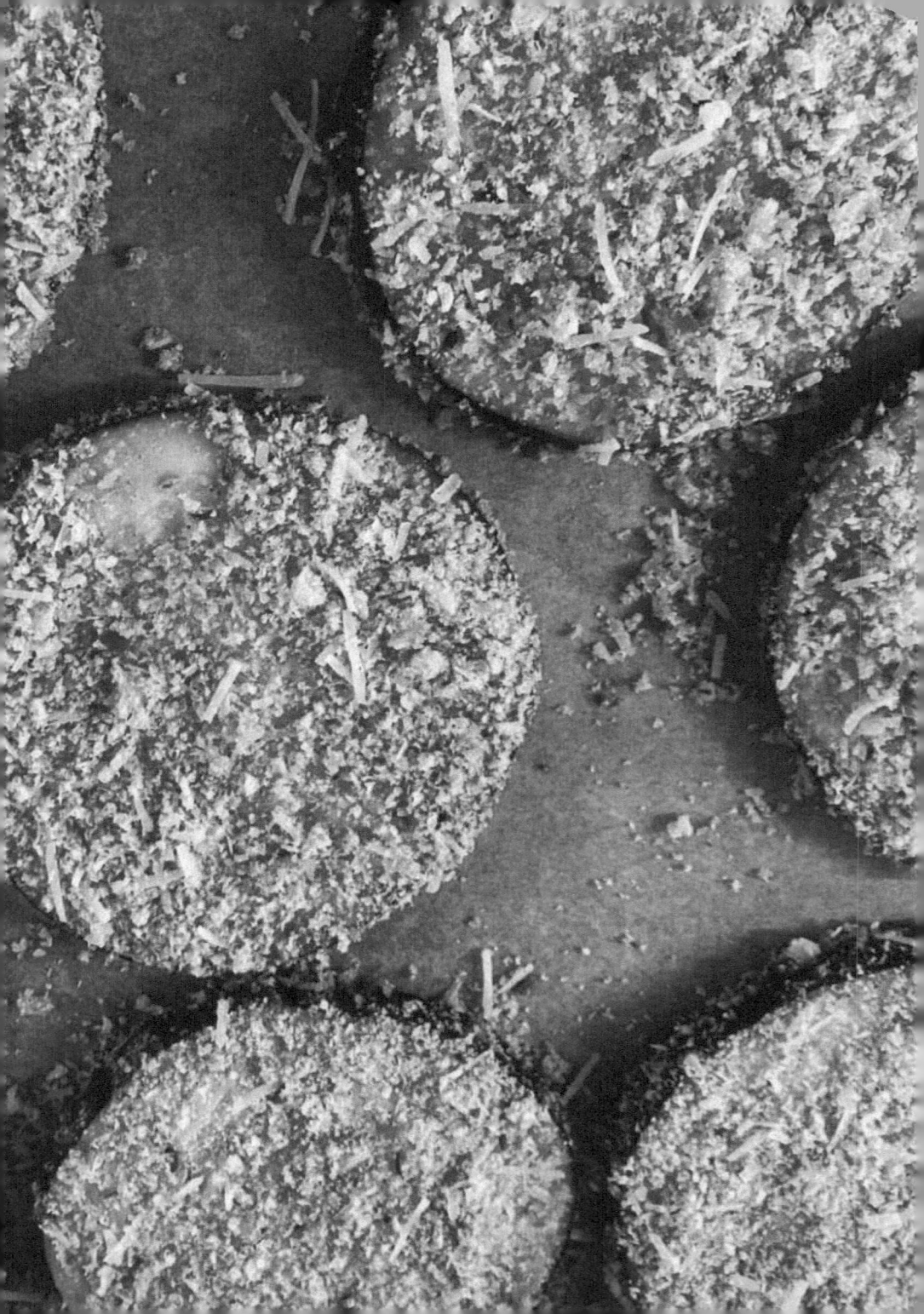

3 week food plan

PANTRY:
Lemons
Limes
Olive oil
Himalayan pink salt
Himalayan herb salt
Almond milk (sugar free)
Oat milk (sugar free)
Sunflower oil
Udos oil
Vegetable bullion powder
Honey
Almonds
Dried fruit
Herbal teas
Eggs
Juicing machine
Smoothie machine
Parchment paper

*Please note: recipes are for 1.
You can easily adapt ingredients for more servings.*

*For a quick and easy dressing, squeeze on a lemon or lime
and add a little udos oil and pink salt on any dish.*

*Some days will be more cooking than others.
I have tried to spread it out evenly through the weeks.*

Always bake with sunflower oil and use olive oil for cold only.

Don't forget to drink plenty of filtered water.

week 1

Breakfast 7am
Oatmeal

1 cup of oatmeal with almond milk

Shopping list:
Packet of milled oatmeal
Raisins
Almond milk

Instructions:
(follow cooking instructions on packet)
Garnish with ½ cup of raisins.
(You can add a little cold water if too thick)
Cook on a medium heat for about 25 minutes stir frequently

Snack 11am
Banana smoothie

Shopping list
1 banana
1 mango (flesh)
2 cups of coconut water
1 spoon full of udos oil (follow guidelines on packet)

Instructions:
Blend together in a smoothie maker/blender

Lunch 1pm
Avocado on buckwheat toast

Shopping list
1 large Avocado
1 Lemon to squeeze over
Himalayan herb salt
Buckwheat bread loaf

Instructions
Cut the Avocado down the middle and wiggle out the stone.
Scoop out the flesh and spread on the toast.
Squeeze the lemon over and add Himalayan salt to taste.

day 1

Snack 4pm
Almond butter oat cake with a bunch of red grapes.

Shopping list:
Oat cakes
Organic Almond butter
Red grapes

Instructions:
Spread the Almond butter on 3 oat cakes and enjoy with the grapes.

Dinner 7pm
Stuffed red peppers with feta and brown rice.

Shopping list:
2 Red peppers
1 cup of brown rice
80g of feta cheese
1 Baby gem lettuce
½ cucumber
½ defrosted sweetcorn
1 lemon

Instructions:
Set oven at 160 c
Cut the tops off the peppers and clean out the seeds inside.
Sprinkle with a little sunflower oil and pop on a baking tray.
Place in oven for 15 minutes.
Meanwhile bring to boil the rice in a litre of water (you can add a teaspoon of bullicn powder to make a vegetable stock) then cover and simmer for about 20 minutes.
Drain any leftover water from rice and stuff into the peppers, crumble the feta on the top then place the tops back on.
Put back in the oven for a further 2 minutes.
Serve with salad and a squeeze of lemon juice.

week 1

Breakfast 7.30 am
Nutty granola with Oat milk

Shopping list:
1 cup of jumbo oats
2 table spoons of honey
½ cup of almonds
1 cup of raw pumpkin seeds
3 table spoons of olive oil
½ cup of dried dates

Instructions:
Oven 160c
Bring to the boil 1 pint of water and add the dates.
Simmer for about 10 minutes.
With the dates, add all the other ingredients, spread out on a parchment covered baking tray. Drizzle the honey over the top and bake for 30 minutes.
When cooled transfer into an air tight container, this will last the week.

Snack 11am
Green smoothie

Shopping list:
1 ripe pear
Bunch of Kale
Bunch of mint
1 apple
1 cup of filtered water
1 spoonful of udos oil

Instructions:
Chop up all items and juice in the juicer.

Lunch 1pm
1 left over red stuffed pepper from yesterday with a green salad

Shopping list:
1/4 Iceberg lettuce
¼ cucumber
1 spoonful of organic plain sauerkraut

day 2

Instructions:
Eat cold as a salad
Shred the lettuce and mix through the sauerkraut with the chopped-up cucumber, add as a side dish to the pepper, season with pink salt.

Snack 4pm
Hummus with celery

Shopping list:
Celery
Bought tub of organic hummus (or homemade)

Instructions:
Wash and trim celery, on a plate spoon 2 large dollops of humus and dip in with celery!
Enjoy

Dinner 7pm
Raw courgette pasta with tofu kebabs.

Shopping list:
1 large courgette
1 red onion
1 red or yellow pepper
80g tofu
1 lemon
1 table spoon of olive oil

Instructions:
Shred the courgette with a vegetable peeler into thin slices.
Chop the tofu, onion and pepper into 1 Inch chunks.
Push them onto a wooden kebab stick then rub on a little sunflower oil and cook on a griddle for a few minutes each side until tofu is slightly golden.
Squeeze the lemon and add the olive together (season with pink salt to taste)
Mix together and pour over the courgette.
Enjoy!
(Make a little extra for tomorrows lunch).

week 1

Breakfast 7am
Oatmeal with Kefir & Honey.

Shopping list:
1 small bottle of organic plain kefir
Oatmeal ref: (day 1)
Almond milk
Honey

Instructions:
Cook Oatmeal to packet instructions with the almond milk
Transfer to bowl and pour 2 large spoonfuls of kefir over the oats then drizzle 1 teaspoon of honey on top.

Snack 11am
1 handful of almonds and dried apricots.

Lunch 1pm
Left over Kebabs and courgette from yesterdays dinner. Eat hot or cold (optional).

Snack 4pm
Kefir, strawberry and banana smoothie.

Shopping list:
1 banana
1 small bottle of kefir
1 handful of large strawberries
1 spoonful of udos oil

Instructions:
Chop up all the fruit, then pour in the kefir and udos oil,
Blend in smoothie maker until smooth.
Enjoy!

day 3

Dinner 7pm
My favourite braised fennel with poached salmon.

Shopping list:
2 line caught salmon steaks
1 large fennel bulb
2 cups of green lentils
Vegetable bullion powder
1 teaspoon on sunflower oil
(keep some for tomorrows lunch)

Instructions:
Oven 160c
Wash and slice the fennel into 8 stripes
Sprinkle over the oil
Bake for 15 minutes.
Mix 1 teaspoon of bullion powder with half a pint of water.
Take the fennel out of the oven and place the fish (skin side up) then pour the stock over.
Pop back in the oven for another 15 minutes.

Meanwhile bring to boil the lentils, then simmer for 20 minutes or until they are soft.

Drain the lentils and place them on a plate and serve the fish, stock and fennel piled up.

Enjoy!

week 1

Breakfast 7am
Granola with Almond milk.

Shopping list:
Almond milk
Granola from day 2

Instructions:
2 cups of homemade granola
Add 2 cups of almond milk

Snack 11am
Oat cakes with almond butter.

Shopping list:
3 oat cakes
Almond butter
5 dried apricots

Instructions:
Spread the butter on the oat cakes and eat with the apricots.

Lunch 1pm
Sweet baked potato with feta

Shopping list:
1 medium sweet potato
80g feta cheese
¼ cup of pitted green olives
¼ cucumber
Half an avocado

Instructions:
Oven !80c
Bake the potato for about 35 minutes until soft
Meanwhile chop up the cucumber and avocado and place in bowl.
Crumble the feta and scatter the olives & mix together.
Take the potato out of the oven and cut open, Place the salad inside.
Enjoy.

day 4

Snack 4pm
Peach smoothie

Shopping list:
1 large peach
1 banana
2 cups of almond milk
Udos oil

Instructions:
Take the stone out of the peach and cut up
Blend all the ingredients together until smooth.

Dinner 7pm
Portobello mushroom with fennel coleslaw.

Shopping list:
2 large portobello mushroom
1 large carrot
1 fennel bulb
1 red onion
20g of hard goat cheese
1 large spoonful of oat yogurt
1 lemon
Pinch of pink salt
(keep 1 portion for tomorrows lunch)

Instructions:
Oven 180c
Wash and place the mushroom on a baking tray.
Bake for 10 minutes
Take out then grate the cheese on the top and place back in for 8 minutes.

Meanwhile…
Thinly slice up all the veggies and place in a bowl, stir in the yogurt, squeeze in the lemon and add a pinch of salt.

Plate up together with the mushroom.
Enjoy!

week 1

Breakfast 7am
Oatmeal

Shopping list:
! cup of oatmeal
2 cups of oat milk

Instructions:
Cook oatmeal to packet instructions with the Oat milk on a medium heat.

Snack 11am
Fennel, apple and avocado smoothie.

Shopping list:
1 avocado (stone removed)
1 small fennel bulb
1 large green apple
1 spoon full of udos oil

Instructions:
Juice the apple and fennel then transfer the juice to the smoothie maker. Add the flesh of the avocado and udos oil. Blend till smooth.

Lunch 1pm
Yesterdays dinner (mushroom and slaw) heat in oven for a 10 mins at 180c or eat cold.

Snack 4pm
Handful of almonds and a piece of sliced apple.

day 5

Dinner 7pm
Butternut squash salad.

Shopping list:
1 large butternut squash
1 cup of green lentils
1 cup of brown rice
Mixed seeds
2 table spoons of Tamari paste

Instructions:
oven 180c
Roast the squash for 35 mins
Scoop out the flesh and cut into cubes.
Boil the lentils for 20 minutes and add ingredients together.
Meanwhile put the seeds on some parchment paper and add the tamari paste, bake in the oven for 10 minutes then sprinkle oven the lentils and squash.
Serve with a green side salad.

week 1

Breakfast 7am
Homemade granola with Plant based milk of choice. (ref: day 2)

Snack 11am
A big red apple and handful of nuts

Lunch 1pm
Goats halloumi with brown rice salad.

Shopping list:
80g of Goats halloumi
1 cup of brown rice
Bullion powder

Instructions:
Grill the sliced halloumi for 5 minutes each side.
Meanwhile bring to boil the rice, add I tea spoon of bullion powder and simmer for 30 minutes (check packet)
Serve with steamed broccoli and salad.

Snack 4pm
Green juice

Shopping list:
1 cucumber
1 apple
½ fennel
handful of mint
udos oil

Instructions:
Chop up and juice all ingredients in a juicer add 1 spoon full of udos oil.

day 6

Dinner 7pm
Noodle salad

Shopping list:
100g buck wheat noodles
80g defrosted cooked edamame beans
150g broccoli
1 table spoon of sesame seeds
1 spring onion
Handful of coriander
1 lemon
2 table spoons of olive oil
Salt to taste

Instructions:
Oven 180c

Cook noodles as instructed on packet
Bake the broccoli in the oven for 10 minutes
Chop the onion and add all together.
Add the beans in a bowl with the cooked noodles then
Lastly add the seeds and enjoy.

week 1

Breakfast 7am
Oatmeal with coconut yogurt

Shopping list:
1 cup of oatmeal
2 table spoons of coconut yogurt
2 cups of almond milk.

Instructions:
Cook oatmeal to packet instructions in almond milk
Place in bowl and add yogurt.

Snack 11am
Handful of mixed seeds and 3 dried apricots

Lunch 1pm
Ploughman oat cakes with tomato salsa

Shopping list:
6 oat cakes
80g of hard Goats cheese
1 tomato
1 spring onion
½ cup of defrosted sweet corn
1 lemon 2 table spoons of olive oil

Instructions:
Slice cheese and place on the oat cakes
Meanwhile in a separate bowl, dice up the salad into 1 Inch cubes and squeeze the lemon and add the oil then mix. Enjoy

Snack 4pm
Molly's super green smoothie

Shopping list:
1 avocado
1 lime
1 handful of basil
1 green apple
1 spoon of udos oil

day 7

Instructions:
De-stone the avocado and place in smoothie maker
Chop and juice all other ingredient then add to smoothie maker and blend all together.
enjoy

Dinner 7pm
Green risotto

Shopping list:
1 tablespoon of sunflower oil
2 cups of risotto rice
1 bunch of asparagus
1 red onion
½ cup of frozen peas
½ bag of rocket
1 teaspoon of Vegetable bullion powder
40g of hard Goats cheese
1 litre of boiling water

Instructions:
Heat the oil in the pan and add the chopped onion. After 5 minutes add the chopped asparagus then add the rice. Meanwhile add boiling water together with the bullion powder in a jug to make a stock. Add a little at a time to the rice mix.
After about 15 minutes it will be cooked.
Before serving add in the rocket and grated cheese then stir through.
(Put two bowls aside for tomorrows lunch and dinner)

Enjoy.

week 2

Breakfast 7am
Homemade Granola with almond milk

Snack 11am
Apple and lime juice with oat cakes.

Shopping list:
3 apples
1 lime
Handful of mint
1 spoon full of udos oil
2 oat cakes
Almond butter
1 table spoon of udos oil

Instructions: spread the almond butter on the oat cakes then juice all other ingredients in the juicer.

Enjoy.

Lunch 1pm
Yesterday's dinner, Risotto. Heat up in a pan on a medium heat for 5 minutes or so and eat with a green salad.

Snack 4pm
1 medium banana.

day 1

Dinner 7pm
Roast butternut squash

Shopping list:
1 medium butternut squash
20g of hard Goats cheese
1 tea spoon of sunflower oil
1 tea spoon of Himalayan herb salt
Small bowl of leftover risotto.

Instructions:
Oven 180c
Cut open the squash long ways down the middle and clean out the seeds.
Score with a knife and drizzle on the oil then rub in the salt
Bake on a baking tray for 35 minutes

Scrape out the flesh and add the mixture to the remaining Risotto from yesterday.
Stuff it all back into the squash and grate on the cheese
Put back in oven for 10 minutes.
Serve with green side salad.

week 2

Breakfast 7am
Oatmeal with chia seeds and honey

Shopping list:
1 cup of oatmeal
2 cups of almond milk
¼ cup of chia seeds
1 tea spoon of honey

Instructions:
Cook oatmeal to packet instructions
5 minutes before the cook time add the chia seeds and honey.

Snack 11am
Strawberry smoothie

Shopping list:
6 strawberries
1 large banana
2 cups of oat milk

Instructions:
Blend together until smooth in a smoothie maker.

Lunch 1pm
Aubergine in cashew pesto.

Shopping list:
1 large Aubergine
2 tablespoons of olive oil
1 teaspoon of sunflower oil
1 handful of coriander
2 cloves of garlic
30g feta
¼ cup of raw cashews

Instructions:
Oven 160c
Slice the aubergine in half longways drizzle with sunflower oil and bake for 25 minutes.

day 2

Meanwhile place all the other ingredients into a blender (except the feta) and blend until smooth and looking like a pesto!

Smooth on the cooked aubergine and sprinkle on the feta.

Enjoy.

Snack 4pm
1 celery stick and a large spoon full of hummus.

Dinner 7pm
Spinach bites in blue corn tacos.

(Because of the amount of lunch prep, here is a nice and simple cheat for tonight).

Shopping list:
1 bag of frozen 'strong roots' spinach bites.
1 packet of blue corn tacos
1 pot of humus
¼ cucumber
Handful of Rocket

Instruction:
Pop 6 bites into the oven and follow packet instructions.
Dry heat the tacos on a pan then add 3 bites in 1 taco
Add some chopped up cucumber and spread some hummus over the bites
Fold up and enjoy using your hands to eat.
Makes 2.
You're welcome.

week 2

Breakfast 7am
Homemade Granola with almond milk.

Snack 11am
Mango smoothie.

Shopping list:
1 medium mango
1 banana
2 cups of coconut water
1 spoonful of udos oil

Instructions:
Remove the stone in the mango, and peel the banana
Blend in a smoothie maker until smooth.

Lunch 1pm
Avocado on toast

Shopping list:
1 medium ripe Avocado
2 slice of buckwheat bread
1 lemon

Instructions:
Remove stone from avocado and spread the flesh onto the toasted buckwheat
Squeeze the lemon over to finish.
Pinch of salt if required.

Snack 4pm
Oat cakes with cheese

Shopping list:
2 oat cakes
2 slices of red apple
20g of hard Goats cheese

Instruction:
Slice the cheese and place on the oat cakes, eat with apple.

day 3

Dinner 7pm
Quinoa and haloumi salad.

Shopping list:
1 cup of quinoa
1 tablespoon of bullion powder
1 fennel bulb
80g of Goats haloumi
1 pepper
1 table spoon of sunflower oil

Instructions:
Oven 170c

Bring a pan of water to the boil then add the quinoa (follow packet instructions)
Add the bullion powder and whisk in (to make vegetable stock)
Meanwhile slice the fennel into 6 long pieces and de-seed the pepper, cut into 4.
Place the fennel and pepper together and
Sprinkle on the oil, bake on a parchment covered tray for 15 minutes
Drain any excess water from the quinoa and mix together with the roasted veg.
(put some quinoa aside for tomorrows dinner)

Cut the goats haloumi and grill for 5 minutes each side.

Serve piled up on top of the salad.

Enjoy.

week 2

Breakfast 7am
Fruit salad

Shopping list:
Any leftover fruit in the fridge chopped up
2 table spoons of oat yogurt
1 spoonful of Mixed seeds to garnish

Snack 11am
Raw flaxseed crackers

Shopping list:
Dehydrator sheet
2 large carrots
2 tomatoes
Handful of coriander
½ cup of water
½ lemon juice
Pinch of pink Himalayan salt
20g of pre soaked (2 hours) flax seeds.

Instructions:
Blend all the ingredients together then add the drained flaxseeds.
Spread the ingredients out thinly onto a dehydrator sheet and dry out for 1 hours.
Break up into crackers and serve on their own or with hummus.

Lunch 1pm
Goats haloumi with pomegranate salad.

Shopping list:
2 spoons of pomegranate seeds
80g of Goats haloumi
1 baby gem lettuce
¼ cucumber
1 spring onion
Handful of spinach leaves
Handful of alfa sprouts

Instructions:
Slice the haloumi into 4 slices and grill each side for 5 minutes. Chops up all the salad and plate up with the haloumi on top. Scatter the pomegranate to finish.

day 4

Snack 4pm
Alkaline regulator juice.

Shopping list:
1 apple
1 fennel bulb
1 beetroot
1 inch of ginger
1 spoonful of udos oil

Instructions:
Chop up and juice in a juicer.

Dinner 7pm
Tuna steak with steamed kale.

Shopping list:
1 table spoon of sunflower oil
1 medium line caught tuna steak
2 handfuls of Kale
Left over quinoa from last night.

Instructions:
Rub the oil over the fish then grill the tuna each side for 5 minutes depending on how much you like it cooked.
Meanwhile, wash and trim the kale and steam it for 7 minutes.
Plate up with some quinoa and season with pink salt.
Enjoy.

week 2

Breakfast 7am
Oatmeal with dried apricots.

Shopping list:
1 cup of oatmeal
2 cups of almond milk
3 dried apricots chopped up

Instructions:
Cook oatmeal to packet instructions with the almond milk then add the apricots.

Snack 11am
Raw flaxseed crackers from yesterday.

Lunch 1pm
Sweet potato with Feta.

Shopping list:
1 medium sweet potato
50g feta
¼ cucumber
Handful of rocket leaves
¼ green pitted olives

Instructions:
Oven 180c
Wash then bake the potato for 35 minutes in the oven
In a bowl mixed the cucumber, olives and rocket together then crumble on the feta.
Cut open the potato and spoon in salad.
Enjoy

Snack 4pm
Apple juice with lime.

Shopping list:
2 apples
½ lime
1 spoonful of udos oil

Instructions:
Chop up fruit and juice in juicer add oil
Enjoy

day 5

Dinner 7pm
Green soup.

Shopping list:
3 sweet potato
1 cup of split peas
1 red onion
2 cloves of garlic
1 teaspoon of bullion powder
1 litre of water
Handful of kale
Handful of Broccoli
1 teaspoon of sunflower oil

Instructions:
Sweat the onion and garlic in a little sunflower oil for 3 minutes
Add the rest of the veg and the water
Whisk in the bullion powder then add the split peas
Bring to boil then simmer for about 30 minutes until the peas are cooked.
Cool down then blend until smooth in a blender.
Eat with left over flaxseed crackers.

week 2

Breakfast 7am
Homemade granola with almond milk.

Snack 11am
Warm almond milk with matcha and oat cake

Shopping list:
1 cup of milk
1 teaspoon of matcha
2 Spoonful of honey
2 oat cakes with honey

Instructions:
Spread the honey on the oat cakes
Warm the milk then add the matcha and stir in the other spoon of honey
Enjoy

Lunch 1pm
Yesterday Green soup

Snack 4pm
Raw flaxseed cracker with hard Goats cheese and red grapes

Shopping list:
Small bunch of grapes
2 crackers
2 slices of cheese

Instructions:
Place cheese on crackers and eat with grapes.

day 6

Dinner 7pm
Falafel with raw fennel coleslaw.

Shopping list:
1 box of falafel kit
1 fennel bulb
3 spring onions
2 carrots
1 lemon
1 spoon of oat yogurt
Instructions:
Cook falafels to the packet instructions

Coleslaw:
Thinly and roughly chop all the veg then in a bowl add the yogurt and squeeze in the lemon juice, then mix together.
Serve a cup full with 4 or 5 Falafel
enjoy

week 2

Breakfast 7am
Oatmeal

Shopping list:
1 cup of oatmeal
2 cups of oat milk

Instructions:
Follow packet cooking instructions.
Simmer in oat milk.

Snack 11am
Green smoothie

Shopping list:
1 avocado
1 green apple
½ lime
¼ pineapple
1 spoonful of udos oil

Instructions:
Juice the fruit in the juicer then blend it with the smoothie maker along with the avocado and udos.

Lunch 1pm
Mushroom omelette

Shopping list:
1 cup of mushrooms
2 eggs
1 teaspoon of sunflower oil

Instructions:
After washing the mushrooms, slice them up and sauté in the oil for 3 minutes.
Meanwhile, whisk the eggs then add to the pan of mushrooms.
Cook omelette on each side for 3 minutes.

Snack 4pm
Sweet potato brownies!

day 7

Shopping list:
¾ rice flour
¾ cup raw cacao
¼ baking powder
6 oz sweet potato
¾ date syrup
¾ cup Goats butter
1 egg
¼ tea spoon of vanilla extract

Instructions:
Oven 180c
Mix rice flour, baking powder and cacao together in a large bowl.
Meanwhile boil the potato then mash. Add all the ingredients together including the potato melted butter and egg. On some parchment paper, spread out the mixture then bake for 25 minutes. Cool down then cut into 2inch squares.
You're welcome (keep in airtight container for next week!)

Dinner 7pm
Almond crust tart with roasted vegetables

Shopping list:
2 cups of ground almonds
Pinch of pink salt
1 tablespoon of water
1 parsnip
1 beetroot
1 onion
1 tablespoon of sunflower oil
Red pepper
Salad to garnish
Basil to garnish

Instructions:
Pulse the almonds, salt and water together and push into a parchment paper covered oven proof flan dish.
Bake for 25 minutes.
Meanwhile, cut all the veg up into 1-inch squares. Sprinkle on the oil and roast for 25 minutes.
Take out the flan and cool down, then place all the veg inside and garnish with basil.
Serve with green salad.

week 3

Breakfast 7am
Homemade granola with almond milk.

Snack 11am
Handful of nuts and seeds.

Lunch 1pm
Raw courgette pasta with tofu kebabs.

Shopping list:
1 large courgette
1 red onion
1 red or yellow pepper
80g tofu
1 lemon
1 table spoon of olive oil

Instructions:
Shred the courgette with a vegetable peeler into thin slices.
Chop the tofu, onion and pepper into 1 Inch chunks.
Push them onto a wooden kebab stick then rub on a little sunflower oil and cook on a griddle for a few minutes each side until tofu is slightly golden.
Squeeze the lemon and add the olive together (season with pink salt to taste)
Mix together and pour over the courgette.
(make extra for tomorrows lunch)

Snack 4pm
Courgette and kale apple juice.

Shopping list:
1 courgette
Handful of kale
1 apple
1 spoonful of udos oil

Instructions:
Chop up and juice in juicer.

day 1

Dinner 7pm
Feta sweet potato.

Shopping list:
20g of feta
1 sweet potato
¼ cucumber
1 spring onion
1 yellow pepper
¼ cup of green pitted olives
70g of baby spinach
6 tender broccoli stems
½ cup of frozen peas (defrosted)

Instructions:
Oven 180c
Bake the potato for 40 minutes.
Steam the broccoli for 3 minutes then add to a bowl with all the other ingredients chopped into stripes.
Mix together and serve inside the cut open sweet potato.
(save a little salad for tomorrows dinner)

week 3

Breakfast 7am
Strawberry oatmeal

Shopping list:
1 cup of oatmeal
2 cups of oat milk
4 chopped up strawberries

Instructions:
Cook oatmeal in the milk according to the packet instructions.
Add strawberries to garnish.

Snack 11am
Apple juice with oat cakes.

Shopping list:
2 apples
1 spoonful of udos oil
2 oat cakes
3 dried apricots

Instructions:
Chop and juice apples and add oil.
Drink with oat cakes and apricots.
Enjoy

Lunch 1pm
Left over courgette spaghetti from dinner yesterday.

Snack 4pm
Sliced up large red apple with a spoonful of almond butter for dunking!
Enjoy.

day 2

Dinner 7pm
Sweetcorn and bean fritters.

Shopping list:
2 large eggs
1 cup of frozen sweetcorn
½ cup of edamame beans (defrosted)
1 lime
50g rice flour
1 teaspoon of sunflower oil
Handful of coriander

Instructions:
Whisk eggs in large bowl and add flour, coriander, and lime juice then mix together, add all the other ingredients.
In a frying pan add the oil and cook the mixture in small patty type batches. 5 minutes or so each side is enough or until the fritters are slightly golden.
Serve with the feta salad from last night dinner.

week 3

Breakfast 7am
Boiled egg with asparagus soldiers.

Shopping list:
1 egg
asparagus

Instructions:
Pop egg into a pan of cold water and bring to boil. Simmer the egg for 3 minutes.
Grill the asparagus for a few minutes then dip them into the egg yolk.
Enjoy!

Snack 11am
Nectarine smoothie

Shopping list:
1 nectarine
1 banana
1 mango
1 cup of coconut water

Instructions:
Remove the stones then blend everything together in smoothie maker.

Lunch 1pm
Miso Salmon.

Shopping list:
1 spoonful of miso paste
1 line caught salmon filet
Salad for garnish
1 table spoon of sunflower oil

Instructions:
Oven 160c
Sprinkle oil over fish then place in the oven for 15 minutes.
Take out and spread the paste over the fish for another 5 minutes.
Serve with salad of choice.

day 3

Snack 4pm
Handful of seeds and nuts

Dinner 7pm
Spinach, veggie omelette

Shopping list:
2 eggs
Handful of baby spinach
½ red onion
1 teaspoon of sunflower oil
20g hard goat's cheese
½ cup of shiitake mushrooms

Instructions:
Heat oil in a pan on a medium heat and add the onions for 2 minutes. Then add the mushrooms, eggs mixture and spinach. Cook each side for a few minutes or until slightly golden. Then grate on cheese before serving.

week 3

Breakfast 7am
Coconut yogurt with chia seeds.

Shopping list:
½ cup of yogurt
¼ cup of chia seeds
¼ cup of fruit salad

Instructions:
In a bowl mix together
Enjoy

Snack 11am
Handful of seeds and nuts.

Lunch 1pm
Grilled tofu steak

Shopping list:
1 80g tofu steak
5 stems of broccoli

Instructions:
Steam the broccoli for 3 minutes.
Grill the tofu for 5 minutes each side.
Serve with side salad.

Snack 4pm
Beetroot juice

Shopping list:
1 raw beetroot
1 inch of ginger
1 apple
1 carrot
1 spoon of udos oil

Instructions:
Chop up and juice in juicer,

day 4

Dinner 7pm
Baked Goats cheese salad with sweet potato wedges.

Shopping list:
150g Goats cheese
1 large sweet potato
¼ cup green pitted olives
1 spoon of olive oil
1 lemon
Handful of rocket salad leaves

Instructions:
Oven 160c
Chop the potato into wedges and drizzle over the oil.
On a baking tray bake for 20 minutes.
Meanwhile, on parchment paper, place the Goats cheese and bake for 8 minutes.
Serve the cheese placed on the rocket and olives with a side of wedges.
Enjoy

week 3

Breakfast 7am
Oatmeal

Shopping list:
1 cup of oats
2 cups of almond milk
Handful of raisins

Instructions:
Cook according to packet with the milk then add raisins to garnish.

Snack 11am
Fennel and apple juice

Shopping list:
1 medium fennel
1 apple
1 handful
1 spoon of udos oil

Instructions:
Chop and juice in juicer

Lunch 1pm
Almond crust tart with roasted vegetables

Shopping list:
2 cups of ground almonds
Pinch of pink salt
1 tablespoon of water
1 parsnip
1 beetroot
1 onion
1 tablespoon of sunflower oil
Red pepper
Salad to garnish
Basil to garnish

Instructions:
Pulse the almonds, salt and water together and push into a parchment paper covered oven proof flan dish.

day 5

Bake for 25 minutes.
Meanwhile, cut all the veg up into 1-inch squares. Sprinkle on the oil and roast for 25 minutes.
Take out the flan and cool down, then place all the veg inside and garnish with basil. Serve with green salad.

Snack 4pm
Handful of seeds and nuts

Dinner 7pm
Stuffed portobello mushroom with fennel

Shopping list:
2 large portobello mushrooms
2 potatoes
1 parsnip
1 carrot 1 red onion
1 garlic bulb
1 fennel bulb
1 spoon of sunflower oil
1 tea spoon of olive oil.

Instructions:
Oven 160c
Wash the veg and cut up in a rustic style, sprinkle oil over and put in oven for 30 minutes. (cut the potatoes into 1-inch chunks)
Add a pinch of pink salt to taste.
Meanwhile cut the fennel into strips, sprinkle with oil and place on a separate tray. Bake for 10 minutes.
Wash the mushroom and sprinkle with oil, bake for 15 minutes.
Cut the top off the garlic bulb and sprinkle with olive oil, bake for 15 minutes.

(Squeeze the garlic over the mushroom and fennel)

Plate up the mushroom, add the fennel on top and the roasted veggies as a side dish

Enjoy!

week 3

Breakfast 7am
Homemade granola with almond milk.

Snack 11am
Avocado and pineapple smoothie.

Shopping list:
Half a pineapple
1 lime
1 avocado (stone removed)
1 spoon udos oil

Instructions:
Juice the pineapple and lime in a juicer then pour into the smoothie maker along with the avocado and oil.
Blend until smooth.

Lunch 1pm
Noodle salad

Shopping list:
100g buckwheat noodles
80g defrosted cooked edamame beans
150g broccoli
1 table spoon of sesame seeds
1 spring onion
Handful of coriander
1 lemon
2 tablespoons of olive oil
Salt to taste

Instructions:
Oven 180c

Cook noodles as instructed on packet
Bake the broccoli in the oven for 10 minutes
Chop the onion and add all together.
Add the beans in a bowl with the cooked noodles then
Lastly add the seeds and enjoy.

day 6

Snack 4pm
Cheese and oat cakes

Shopping list:
2 oat cakes
Bunch of red grapes
2 slices of hard Goats cheese

Instructions:
Plate up Enjoy

Dinner 7pm
Asparagus and potato and onion frittata

Shopping list:
6 asparagus stems
1 red onion
1 cooked white potato
1 teaspoon on oil
2 eggs
Salad to garnish

Instructions:
Heat oil in pan and add the diced onion, cook for 3 minutes.
Meanwhile peel and boil the potato for 10 minutes.
Remove the potato and chop up into 1-inch pieces.
Add the asparagus and potato to the onions and sauté for 6 minutes.
Add the egg mixture to the veggies and cook for 4 minutes.
Finish off under the grill for a few minutes.
Use a spatula to take out of the pan and plate up with a green salad.

week 3

Breakfast 7am
Homemade Granola with Oat milk.

Snack 11am
Banana and blueberry smoothie

Shopping list:
1 banana
½ cup of blueberry
2 cups of almond milk
1 spoon of udos oil

Instructions:
Blend together in a smoothie maker until smooth.

Lunch 1pm
Tofu steak with sauerkraut and Avocado salad

Shopping list:
½ avocado
1 80g tofu steak
4 asparagus stems
1 large spoon of sauerkraut

Instructions:
Grill the tofu steak and asparagus for 5 minutes each side.
Chop up the avocado and mix with the sauerkraut.
Plate up piled together
Enjoy

Snack 4pm
Sweet potato brownie (leftovers) ref; day 7 week 2

Dinner 7pm
Roasted cauliflower salad

Shopping list:
1 cup of cauliflower
1 roasted parsnip
1 cup of steamed green beans
1 tea spoon of sunflower oil

day 7

Handful of baby spinach
Handful of basil
1 teaspoon of bullion powder
1 tablespoon of Pomegranate pieces
½ cup of green lentils
Pinch of pink salt
Lemon for squeezing

Instructions:
Oven 170c
Wash and cut the cauliflower and parsnip.
Cut them into 1-inch pieces.
Sprinkle with a little oil and Place on a baking tray.
Roast in oven for 20 minutes
Meanwhile, steam the beans for 10 minutes.
Cook the lentils following the packet instructions in a little bullion powder stock.
Pinch of salt to taste.
Squeeze of lemon for taste.

Place all cooked ingredients in a bowl and mix together.

Plate up with a side of spinach and basil

Enjoy

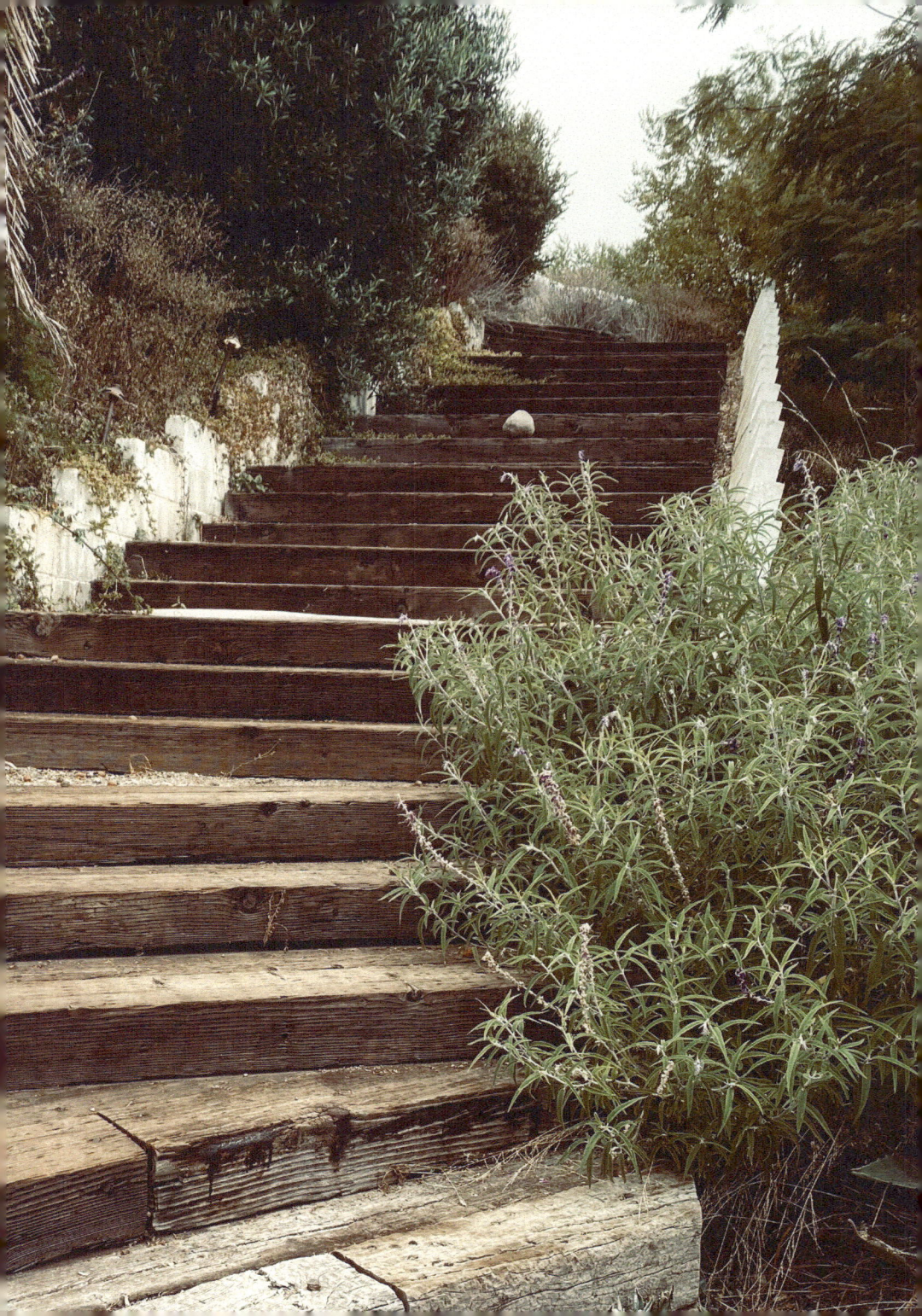

3 week exercise program

YOU WILL NEED:

2kg medicine ball
Pilates ball
Yoga matt
Walking/cross training shoes

Always check with your doctor before exercising

We will be incorporating these key exercises into each week
I have chosen these because they support your core
combined with the walking, this will give you stability and help
with your balance and strength

If you can, try and walk home from work for 10 - 20 minutes a day
Otherwise, please add this into your routine
before the weight bearing exercises

week 1

Day 1

5.45pm
Walk for 10 minutes

6.00pm
Planks: 1 minute x 3 times (1 minute break in between)
Sit-ups (on large yoga ball) slowly raise up and down with hands on ears for 5 x 3 times (1 minute break in between)

Day 2

5.45pm
Walk for 10 minutes

6.00pm
Russian twists (with medicine ball) perch on bottom, with raised legs, and bring ball left to right across your middle, pulling tummy in for 1 minute x 3 times (1 minute break in between)
Abs: (with medicine ball) lying on back, with knees bent, holding ball to chest, sit up then reach to toes, and back down again x 3 (1 minute break in between)

Day 3

5.45pm
Walk for 15 minutes

6.00pm
Bridges: Lying on back, gently raise hips up into bridge position and slowly down again 1 minute x 3 times (1 minute break in between)

Day 4

5.45pm
Walk 10 minutes

6.00pm
Planks: 1 minute x 3 times (1 minute break in between)
Sit-ups (on large yoga ball) slowly raise up and down with hands on ears for 5 x 3 times (1 minute break in between)

Day 5

5.45pm
Walk 15 minutes

6.00pm
Bridges: Lying on back, gently raise hips up into bridge position and slowly down again
1 minute x 3 times (1 minute break in between)

Day 6

5.45pm
Walk for 10 minutes

6.00pm
Russian twists (with medicine ball) perch on bottom, with raised legs, and bring ball left to right across your middle, pulling tummy in for 1 minute x 3 times (1 minute break in between)

Abs: (with medicine ball) lying on back, with knees bent, holding ball to chest, sit up then reach to toes, and back down again x 3 (1 minute break in between

Day 7

5.45pm
Walk 10 minutes

6.00pm
Planks: 1 minute x 3 times (1 minute break in between)
Sit-ups (on large yoga ball) slowly raise up and down with hands on ears for 5 x 3 times (1 minute break in between)

week 2

Day 1

5.45pm
Walk for 15 minutes

6.00pm
Planks: 1 minute x 3 times (1 minute break in between)
Sit-ups (on large yoga ball) slowly raise up and down with hands on ears for 5 x 3 times (1 minute break in between)

Day 2

5.45pm
Walk for 15 minutes

6.00pm
Russian twists (with medicine ball) perch on bottom, with raised legs, and bring ball left to right across your middle, pulling tummy in for 1 minute x 3 times (1 minute break in between)
Abs: (with medicine ball) lying on back, with knees bent, holding ball to chest, sit up then reach to toes, and back down again x 3 (1 minute break in between)

Day 3

5.45pm
Walk for 20 minutes

6.00pm
Bridges: Lying on back, gently raise hips up into bridge position and slowly down again
1 minute x 3 times (1 minute break in between)

Day 4

5.45pm
Walk for 15 minutes

6.00pm
Planks: 1 minute x 3 times (1 minute break in between)
Sit-ups (on large yoga ball) slowly raise up and down with hands on ears for 5 x 3 times (1 minute break in between)

Day 5

5.45pm
Walk for 20 minutes

6.00pm
Bridges: Lying on back, gently raise hips up into bridge position and slowly down again
1 minute x 3 times (1 minute break in between)

Day 6

5.45pm
Walk for 15 minutes

6.00pm
Russian twists (with medicine ball) perch on bottom, with raised legs, and bring ball left to right across your middle, pulling tummy in for 1 minute x 3 times (1 minute break in between)
Abs: (with medicine ball) lying on back, with knees bent, holding ball to chest, sit up then reach to toes, and back down again x 3 (1 minute break in between

Day 7

5.45pm
Walk for 15 minutes

6.00pm
Planks: 1 minute x 3 times (1 minute break in between)
Sit-ups (on large yoga ball) slowly raise up and down with hands on ears for 5 x 3 times (1 minute break in between)

week 3

Day 1

5.45pm
Walk for 20 minutes

6.00pm
Planks: 1 minute x 3 times (1 minute break in between)
Sit-ups (on large yoga ball) slowly raise up and down with hands on ears for 5 x 3 times (1 minute break in between)

Day 2

5.45pm
Walk for 20 minutes

6.00pm
Russian twists (with medicine ball) perch on bottom, with raised legs, and bring ball left to right across your middle, pulling tummy in for 1 minute x 3 times (1 minute break in between)
Abs: (with medicine ball) lying on back, with knees bent, holding ball to chest, sit up then reach to toes, and back down again x 3 (1 minute break in between

Day 3

5.45pm
Walk for 25 minutes

6.00pm
Bridges: Lying on back, gently raise hips up into bridge position and slowly down again
1 minute x 3 times (1 minute break in between)

Day 4

5.45pm
Walk for 20 minutes

6.00pm
Planks: 1 minute x 3 times (1 minute break in between)
Sit-ups (on large yoga ball) slowly raise up and down with hands on ears for 5 x 3 times (1 minute break in between)

Day 5

5.45pm
Walk for 25 minutes

6.00pm
Bridges: Lying on back, gently raise hips up into bridge position and slowly down again
1 minute x 3 times (1 minute break in between)

Day 6

5.45pm
Walk for 20 minutes

6.00pm
Russian twists (with medicine ball) perch on bottom, with raised legs, and bring ball left to right across your middle, pulling tummy in for 1 minute x 3 times (1 minute break in between)
Abs: (with medicine ball) lying on back, with knees bent, holding ball to chest, sit up then reach to toes, and back down again x 3 (1 minute break in between

Day 7

5.45pm
Walk for 20 minutes

6.00pm
Planks: 1 minute x 3 times (1 minute break in between)
Sit-ups (on large yoga ball) slowly raise up and down with hands on ears for 5 x 3 times (1 minute break in between)

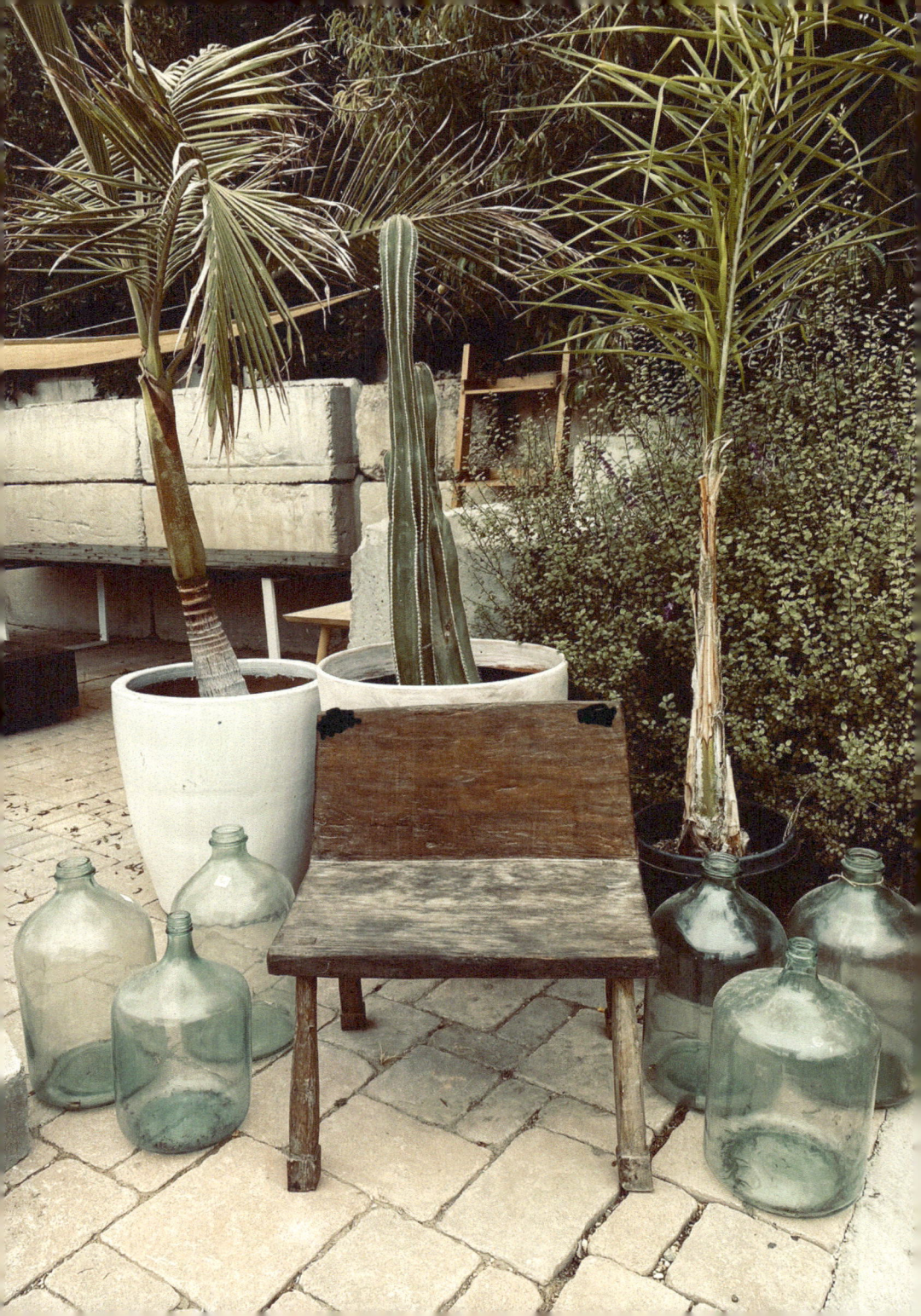

3 week relaxation program

YOU WILL NEED:

Pen
Notebook
Joss sticks
Lavender oil

week 1

Day 1

6.45am

Shopping list:
Note pad (journal)
Pen

On waking, write down whatever comes to mind for 5 minutes
Try not to over think this exercise
Jot down whatever comes to mind
The reason for this is to declutter the mind, so you are then able to think and see more clearly around you
It can be your greatest fears but also your food shopping list
Just write away
You don't need to re-read this, but keep it private

On meditating, keep your eyes
low or close them
Try and be alone and in silence if possible
Lie down or sit up with your spine always straight
Enjoy

Day 2

6.45am

Shopping list:
Joss Sticks

Make notes for 5 minutes
Light Joss Stick and with your eyes closed breathe in for 4 and out for 8 seconds for 1 minute

Day 3

6.45am

Write notes
Light Joss Stick
Breathe in for 4 and out for 8 seconds for 2 minutes

Day 4

6.45am

Make notes
Light Joss Stick
Breathe in for 4 and out for 8 for 3 minutes

Day 5

6.45am

Write notes
Light Joss Stick
Breathe in for 4 and out for 8 seconds for 4 minutes

Day 6

6.45am

Write notes
Light Joss Stick
Breathe in for 5 and out for 10 seconds for 3 minutes

Day 7

6.45am

Write notes
Light Joss Stick
Breathe in for 5 and out for 10 seconds for 4 minutes

week 2

Day 1

6.45am

Write notes
Light Joss Stick
For 3 minutes meditate on your own body (this is called a body scan)
Start at your toes and slowly work towards your head
Slowly breathe in and out

Day 2

6.45am

Write notes
Light Joss Stick
For 3 minutes meditate (body scan)
Toes to head
Focus on your breath when your mind wanders

Day 3

6.45am

Write notes
Light Joss Stick
For 4 minutes meditate (body scan)
Toes to head
Focus on your breath when your mind wanders

Day 4

6.45am

Write notes
Light Joss Stick
For 5 minutes (body scan)
Breathe deep

Day 5

6.45am

Write notes
Light Joss Stick
For 5 minutes (body scan)
Add gentle music
Breathe deep
Enjoy the experience

Day 6

6.45am

Write notes
Light Joss Stick
For 6 minutes (body scan)
Add gentle music
Feel the energy
Breathe deep

Day 7

6.45am

Write notes
Light Joss Stick
For 7 minutes (body scan)
Add music
Breathe in for 5 and out for 10
Picture a light inside of you
Feel the energy

week 3

Day 1

6.45am

Write notes
Light Joss Stick
Change seated position (if you were lying down during body scan, now sit up and close your eyes)
For 8 minutes (body scan)
Add music
Tell yourself to relax deeper

Day 2

6.45am

Write notes
Light Joss Stick
For 8 minutes breathe in for 5 and out for 10
Focus on your breath and belly rising and falling
Feel the energy

Day 3

6.45am

Write notes
Light Joss Stick
For 9 minutes very slowly (body scan)
Add gentle music

Day 4

6.45am

Write notes
Light Joss Stick
(you should be in a relaxation habit now)
Breathe deeply in for 6 (if you can) and out for 9
10 minutes

Day 5

6.45am

Write notes
Light Joss Stick
Body scan for 10 minutes
Add gentle music
Focus on the belly rising and falling
Enjoy

Day 6

6.45am

Write notes
Light Joss Stick
Body scan for 10 minutes
With a little lavender oil in hand, you can finish by gently massaging your neck for 1 minute

Day 7

6.45am

Write notes
Light Joss Stick
Breathe deep for 5 seconds in and 10 seconds out for 10 minutes
Focus on the belly rising and falling
Add relaxation music
Finish with massaging your neck and shoulders with a little lavender for 2 minutes

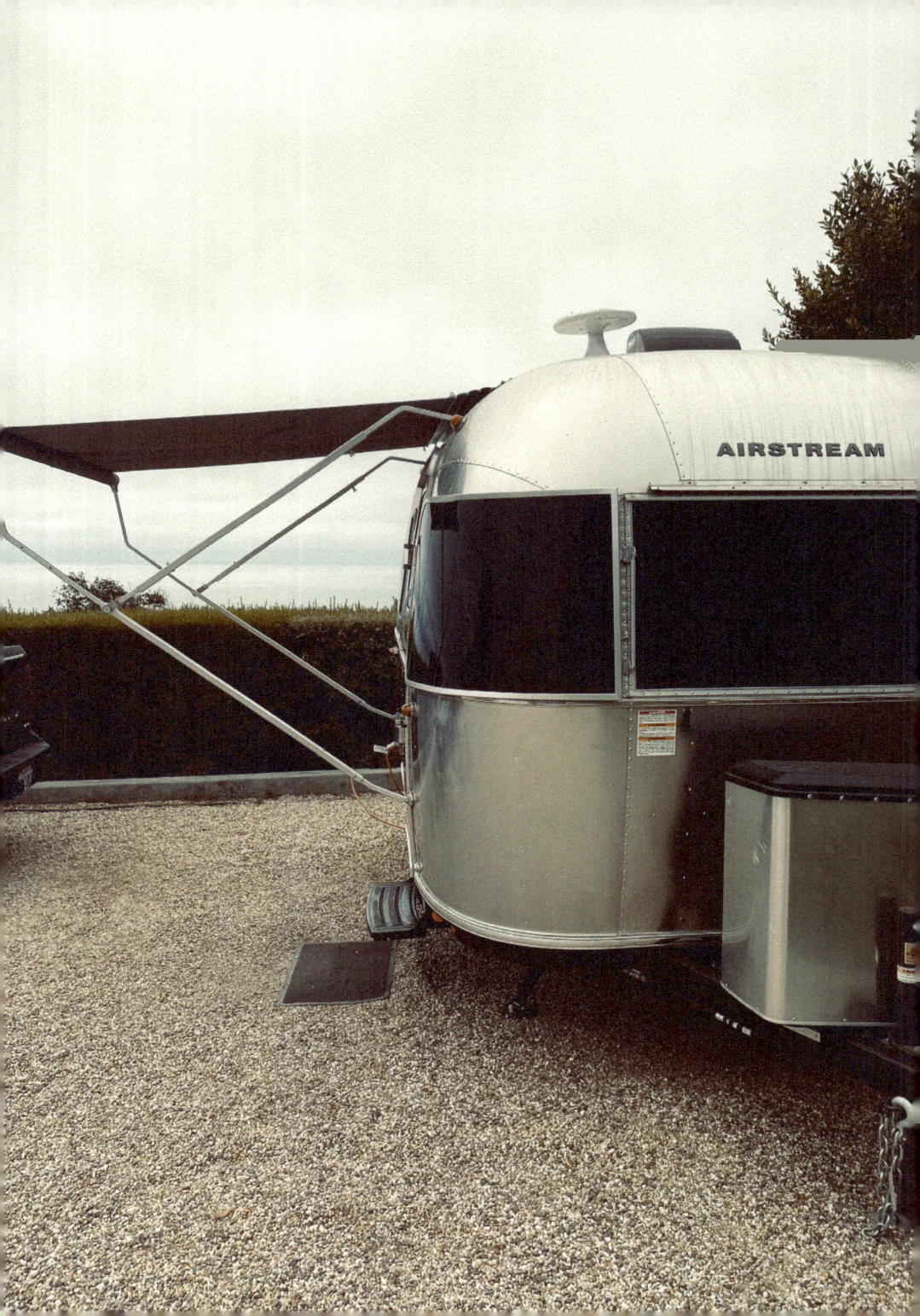

notes

notes

notes

notes

notes

notes

notes

notes

notes

notes

notes

notes

notes

notes

notes

notes

First published 2023

Copyright © Emma Lehane 2023

The right of Emma Lehane to be identified as the author of this work has been asserted in accordance with the Copyright, Designs & Patents Act 1988.

All rights reserved. No part of this book may be reproduced, stored in a retrieval system, or transmitted in any form or by any means, electronic, electrostatic, magnetic tape, mechanical, photocopying, recording or otherwise, without the written permission of the copyright holder.

Published under licence by Brown Dog Books,
10b Greenway Farm, Bath Rd, Wick nr. Bath BS30 5RL

ISBN printed book: 978-1-83952-749-4

All images ©2023 by Emma Lehane
Book design by www.lollipop-studio.co.uk

Printed and bound in the UK

emma.alkalineway@gmail.com

This book is printed on FSC® certified paper

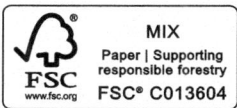

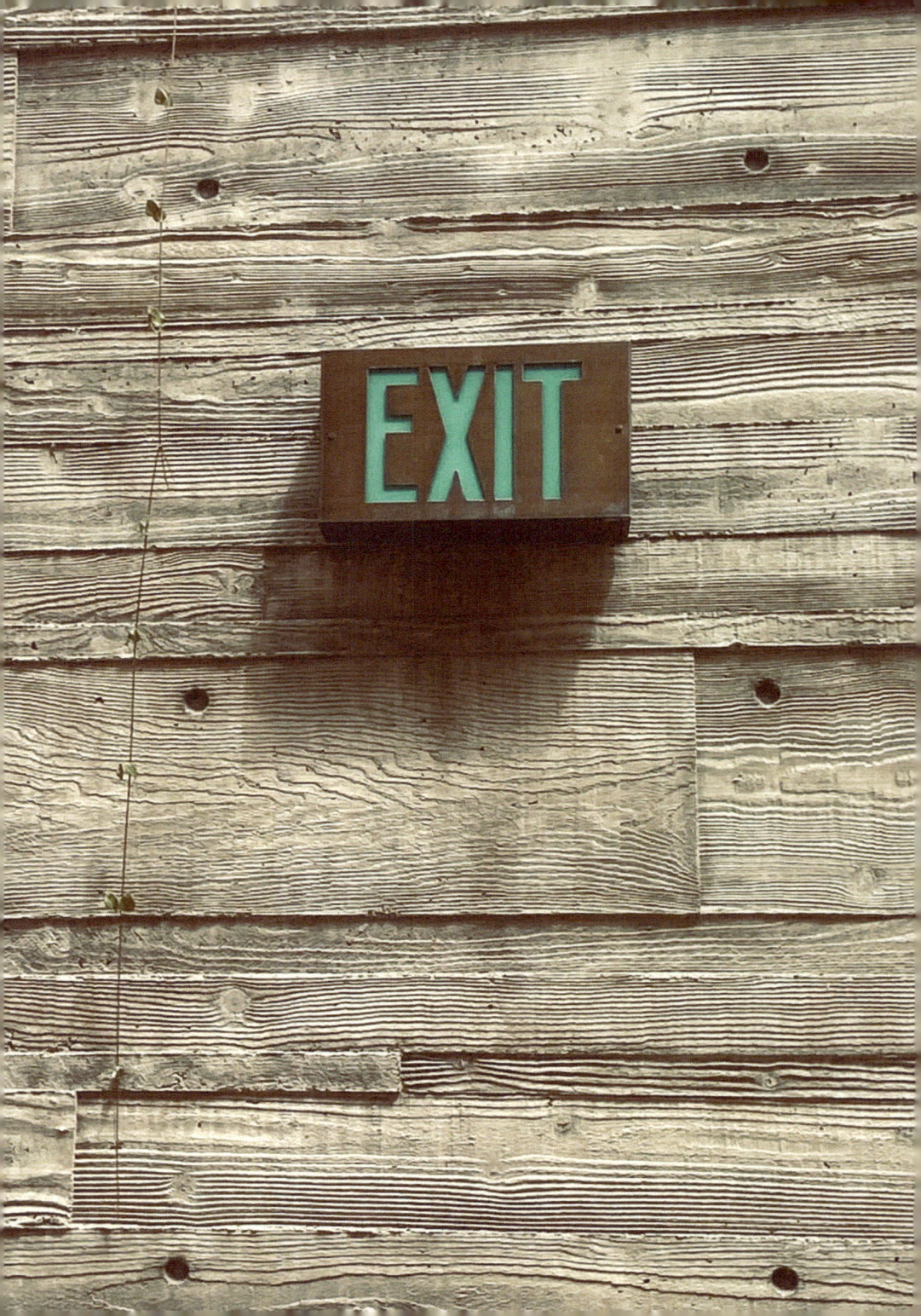